PALEO GUT HEALTH COOKBOOK

Gut Friendly Recipes and Meal Plan to Restore Digestive Balance and Boost Well-Being

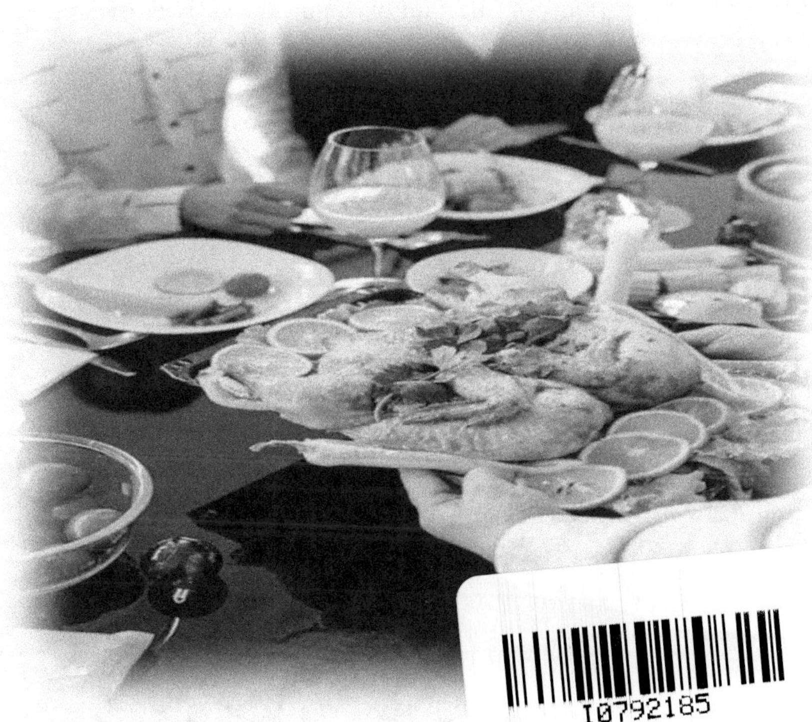

CHRISTIANA WHITE

GAIN ACCESS TO MORE BOOKS

TABLE OF CONTENTS

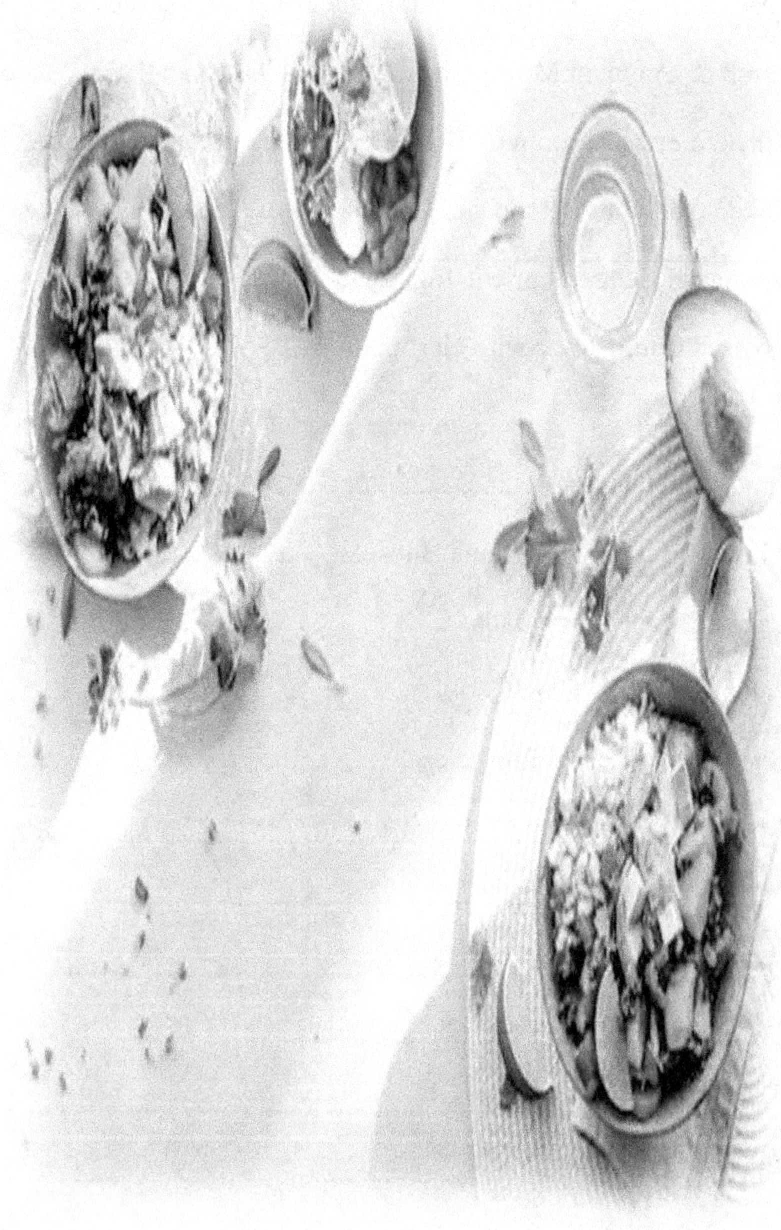

INTRODUCTION

Do you experience digestive symptoms such as bloating, gas, constipation, diarrhea, or pain? Do you always feel weary, moody, or inflamed? Do you have allergies, autoimmune diseases, or other chronic health issues? If you responded yes to any of the above questions, this book is for you.

This book is more than just a cookbook. It is a handbook that will help you heal your stomach and restore your health using Paleo principles. Paleo is not a trendy diet. It is a manner of eating based on the foods that our forefathers ate for millions of years before the introduction of agriculture, industrialization, and processed foods. Paleo does not involve counting calories, carbohydrates, or points. It is about consuming real, healthy, natural meals that nourish both your body and mind.

But Paleo isn't enough. If you have a damaged or leaky gut, you must take additional efforts to repair and support your digestive system. That's why this book introduces you to the Paleo gut healing diet, which blends Paleo principles with cutting-edge scientific research into gut health.

This book will teach you how to follow the Paleo gut healing diet and prepare delicious and easy foods that will help you feel and look amazing.

You'll also find Paleo gut healing meal and snack tips and techniques, commonly asked questions and common myths about the Paleo gut healing diet, as well as resources and references for further information and support.

This book is based on my personal experience as well as the experiences of many others who have tried the Paleo gut healing diet and seen incredible benefits. I've been following the Paleo gut healing diet for more than a year and have never felt healthier.

I've mended my stomach, cured my autoimmune disease, reduced weight, enhanced my skin, and rediscovered my vitality and joy. I've also helped many of my clients and friends get similar results with the Paleo gut healing diet.

I produced this book to share my expertise and passion with you, as well as to assist you in healing your gut and transforming your health through Paleo principles. I hope this book inspires, motivates, and empowers you to take control of your health and well-being. I hope this book will be a helpful companion and guide on your path to Paleo gut healing.

Thank you for choosing this book and entrusting me to assist you. I appreciate your support and wish you the best. Let's get started.

CHAPTER 1

Overview of the Paleo Gut Healing Diet.

The Paleo gut healing diet is a style of eating that tries to repair and support your digestive system's health by adhering to Paleo diet principles while avoiding foods that can cause inflammation, allergies, or autoimmune reactions.

The Paleo gut healing diet can help you reduce bloating, gas, constipation, diarrhea, and other digestive symptoms, improve nutrient absorption and assimilation, boost immune system function and lower your risk of infection, reduce inflammation and pain in the body, balance hormones and mood, and increase energy and vitality.

The Paleo gut healing diet focuses on foods that are nutrient-dense, anti-inflammatory, and easy to digest, such as:

- Meat, poultry, fish, and eggs from pastured, organic, or wild sources.
- Seasonal, organic vegetables and fruits.
- Healthy fats include coconut oil, olive oil, avocado, ghee, and animal fats.
- Nuts and seeds, preferably sprouted.
- Fermented foods include sauerkraut, kimchi, kombucha, and coconut yogurt.

- Bone broth, gelatin, collagen
- Herbs and spices including ginger, turmeric, garlic, rosemary, and cinnamon.

You should also avoid foods that can harm your gut lining, create inflammation, or activate immunological responses, such as:

- Grains include wheat, rice, corn, oats, and quinoa.
- Legumes: beans, peas, lentils, and soy.
- Dairy, including milk, cheese, yogurt, and butter.
- Sugars and artificial sweeteners.
- Processed and refined foods, including bread, spaghetti, cereal, chips, and cookies
- Vegetable oils: canola, soybean, corn, and sunflower oil.
- Alcohol and Caffeine
- Nightshade veggies, including tomatoes, potatoes, peppers, and eggplants (for certain people).
- Eggs, nuts, seeds, and spices (for some patients with autoimmune diseases).

The Paleo gut healing diet is not a one-size-fits-all solution. You may need to tailor it to your specific needs, interests, and goals. You may also want to experiment with different foods to see how they effect your gut and overall health.

The Paleo gut healing diet is not severe or restrictive. It is a flexible and adaptable diet that allows you to enjoy a wide range of foods and flavors as long as they are beneficial to your stomach and overall health.

Importance of Gut Health

Your gut health is critical not only for digestion, but also for your general health and wellbeing. Your gut contains trillions of bacteria, collectively known as the gut microbiome, that conduct a variety of roles, including:

- Digestion and breakdown of complex carbs, proteins, and lipids.
- Manufacturing vitamins including vitamin K, B12, B9, and biotin.
- Controlling metabolism and altering weight and body composition.
- Improving immunity and safeguarding against infections and poisons.
- Influencing mood and brain function via generating neurotransmitters like serotonin and dopamine.
- Protecting against inflammation and oxidative stress by creating short-chain fatty acids like butyrate and propionate.

Numerous things influence your gut health, including:

- Your diet, including the quality and variety of the meals you consume.
- Your lifestyle, including the quantity and quality of your sleep, exercise, and stress management.
- Your drugs, including antibiotics, steroids, NSAIDs, and birth control pills.
- Infections and exposure to pathogens such bacteria, viruses, fungi, and parasites.
- Your genetics and hereditary factors that influence gut microbiota makeup and function.
- Your environmental exposures and the contact with chemicals, pollutants, and poisons

Your gut health can also affect several elements of your health, such as:

- Your immune system and your vulnerability to infections, allergies, and autoimmune illnesses
- Your inflammation and your risk of chronic diseases, such as diabetes, cardiovascular disease, and cancer
- Your hormones and your reproductive health, fertility, and monthly cycle
- Your mood and your mental health, such as depression, anxiety, and cognitive decline

- Your skin health and your appearance, such as acne, eczema, and psoriasis

- Your weight and your appetite, fullness, and cravings

Therefore, maintaining a healthy and balanced gut is vital for your maximum health and well-being.

Impact of Diet on Gut Health

Your food is one of the most critical elements that affect your gut health. What you eat can either nourish or destroy your gut microbiota, and subsequently, your health.

Eating foods that are nutrient-dense, anti-inflammatory, and simple to digest will assist you:

- Support and diversify your gut microbiome and increase the beneficial bacteria, such as Bifidobacteria and Lactobacilli

- Heal your gut lining and seal any leaks that trigger inflammation and immunological reactions.

- Improve your digestive function and enhance your nutrient absorption and assimilation

- Reduce inflammation and pain in the body and joints.

- Boost your immune system and lower your risk of infections and autoimmune diseases

- Balance your hormones and mood, and improve your mental clarity and attention.
- Boost your energy and vigor while helping you lose weight and maintain a healthy body composition.

Eating foods that are nutrient-poor, inflammatory, and hard to digest can damage your gut microbiome, and cause:

- Dysbiosis and imbalance of your gut microbiome and decrease the beneficial bacteria, such as Bifidobacteria and Lactobacilli
- Leaky gut and increased permeability of your gut lining that allows toxins and pathogens to enter your bloodstream
- Impaired digestive function and reduced nutrient absorption and assimilation
- Increased inflammation and pain in your body and joints
- Compromised immune system and higher risk of infections and autoimmune diseases
- Imbalanced hormones and mood and impaired mental clarity and focus
- Decreased energy and vitality and weight gain and obesity

Therefore, choosing the right foods for your gut health is crucial for your health and well-being.

CHAPTER 2

Essential Kitchen Tools and Ingredients

To follow the Paleo gut healing diet, you will want certain basic kitchen utensils and materials to make cooking easier and more fun. Here are some of the essential goods you will require:

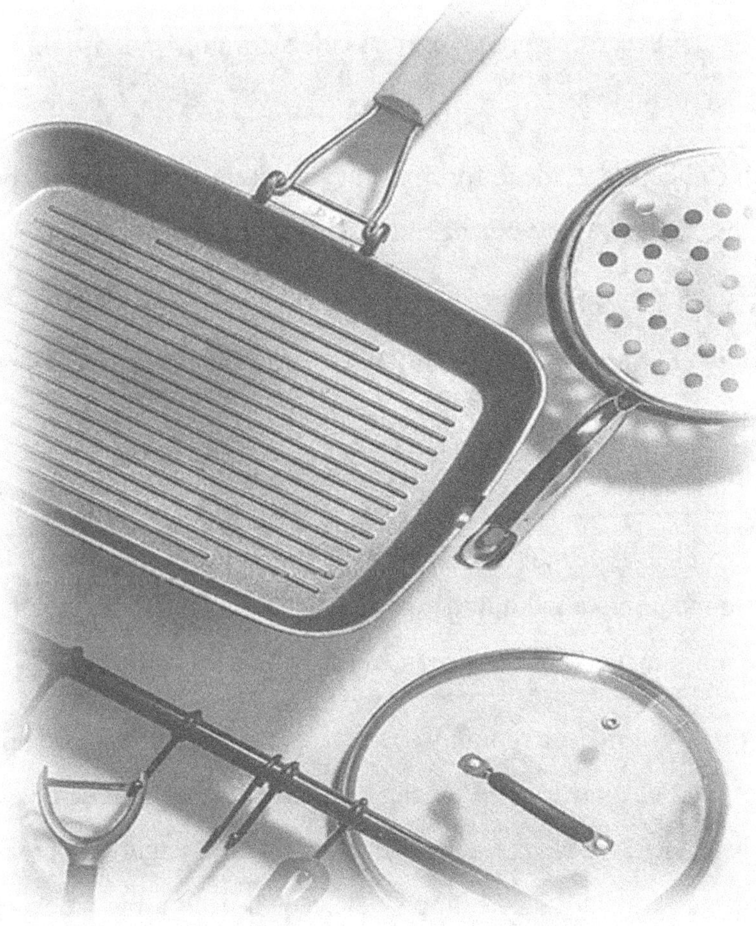

• **A decent pair of knives and a chopping board**. You'll be slicing a lot of vegetables, fruits, meat, and herbs, so sharp, strong blades and a large, steady cutting board are essential. You can also get a food processor or blender to create sauces, soups, smoothies, and purees.

• **A cast-iron skillet and baking sheet**. These are multipurpose cooking equipment that can be used to prepare meat, fish, eggs, veggies, and even dessert. Cast iron skillets are sturdy, nonstick, and can tolerate high heat.

Baking sheets are ideal for roasting, broiling, and baking. For simpler cleanup, line your baking sheets with parchment paper or silicone mats.

• **A slow cooker and an Instant Pot**. These are useful appliances that can help you save time and effort. They can be used to prepare soft and tasty meat, soups, stews, and bone broth.

You can also use them to cook grains, beans, and potatoes if you want to incorporate them into your diet. You may put them together in the morning and have a nice meal ready by the evening.

• **A stockpot and saucepan**. These are great for preparing soups, sauces, and heating water. You can even utilize them to create your own fermented foods like sauerkraut, kimchi, and yogurt. To create bone broth, a Paleo gut-healing staple, you'll need a big stockpot.

You'll also need a pot to melt coconut oil, ghee, or butter and heat up liquids.

• **Salad spinner and colander.** These are ideal for washing and drying leafy greens, herbs, and other vegetables. They can also be used to drain and rinse nuts, seeds, and grains before soaking and sprouting them.

A salad spinner can also help you drain extra water from cooked veggies like cauliflower or zucchini before cooking rice or noodles with them.

• **A measuring cup and spoon**. These are required for measuring your ingredients, particularly when following recipes. You can also use them to measure oil, vinegar, and other liquids while making dressings and marinades. Dry and liquid measurement cups can be used separately or together. If you want, you can weigh your items on a kitchen scale.

• **Spatula, whisk, and wooden spoon.** These are the fundamental utensils you'll need for stirring, flipping, scraping, and mixing food. A spatula is used for flipping pancakes, eggs, and burgers, as well as scraping the sides of a skillet or baking dish.

A whisk is useful for beating eggs, whipping cream, and emulsifying dressings. A wooden spoon can be used to stir soups, sauces, and casseroles to keep them from sticking or burning.

• **A Mason jar and a glass container**. These are ideal for keeping your handmade fermented foods, bone broth, sauces, and dressings. You may also use them to keep leftovers, snacks, and salads. Mason jars are perfect for fermenting because their tight cover keeps air from entering while allowing gas to leave.

Glass containers are preferred over plastic ones because they are more durable, environmentally friendly, and do not leach toxins into your food.

In addition to these culinary items, you will require several fundamental ingredients that are typical in the Paleo gut healing diet, such as:

• **Coconut oil, olive oil, avocado oil, ghee, and animal fat.** These are healthy fat sources that are anti-inflammatory, easy to digest, and full of flavor. You can use them to cook, bake, or season your cuisine.

Coconut oil is especially advantageous since it contains antibacterial qualities that can help battle harmful bacteria and yeast in your gut. Ghee is clarified butter that has been cooked and strained to eliminate milk particles, making it appropriate for dairy-sensitive individuals.

• **Sea salt, black pepper, garlic, onion, ginger, turmeric, rosemary, thyme, oregano, basil, parsley, cilantro, and more**

herbs and spices. These are natural taste enhancers that can make your food both delicious and wholesome. They also have a variety of health benefits, including improved digestion, reduced inflammation, increased immunity, and ability to fight infections.

Garlic, onion, ginger, and turmeric are particularly effective because to their antibacterial, antifungal, and anti-inflammatory characteristics, which can aid in gut healing.

Rosemary, thyme, oregano, basil, parsley, and cilantro are also high in antioxidants, vitamins, and minerals, which can benefit your health.

• **Apple cider vinegar, lemon juice, lime juice, and other acidic beverages.** These can be used to flavor and brighten your food, as well as help preserve and ferment it. They can also help with digestion by increasing the production of stomach acid and bile, both of which are necessary for food breakdown and nutritional absorption.

They can also assist to regulate your pH and inhibit the formation of dangerous bacteria and yeast in your gut.

• **Natural sweeteners including honey, maple syrup, and coconut sugar.** These are optional, although they can lend a hint of sweetness to your cuisine, particularly sweets and beverages. You should use them rarely since they contain sugar, which can feed harmful bacteria and yeast in your gut, causing inflammation and blood sugar increases.

You should also avoid artificial sweeteners like aspartame, sucralose, and saccharin, which can alter your gut microbiota and create a variety of health issues.

• **Dark chocolate, dried fruits, nuts, and seeds**. These are optional, but they can help add crunch, chew, and richness to your cuisine, particularly snacks and sweets. You can also utilize them to make nut and seed butters, milks, flours, and oils that can be used in place of dairy and gluten in recipes.

To minimize antinutrients and enhance digestion, choose raw, unsalted, and organic nuts and seeds, then soak and sprout them before consuming.

To avoid additional sugar and chemicals, choose unsweetened, sulfite-free, organic dried fruits, as well as dark chocolate with at least 70% cocoa.

Foods to Include and Avoid.

To follow the Paleo gut healing diet, you must include and avoid particular foods based on their impact on your gut and overall health. Here are some of the foods you should eat and avoid:

Foods to Include:

• **Meat, poultry, fish, and eggs from pastured, organic, or wild animals.** These are high-quality protein sources that are necessary for the development and repair of your tissues, including the gut wall. They also contain nutrients such as iron, zinc, selenium, B vitamins, and omega-3 fatty acids, which are beneficial to your health and well-being.

You should consume lean meats, skinless chicken, and low-mercury fish, and avoid processed meats like bacon, ham, sausage, and deli meats, which are heavy in salt, nitrates, and preservatives and can harm your gut and raise your risk of cancer.

• **Organic or seasonal vegetables and fruits.** These are high-fiber foods that can help feed your beneficial bacteria and support regular bowel motions. They also contain a variety of vitamins, minerals, antioxidants, and phytochemicals that can protect your cells from harm, reduce inflammation, and boost your immune system.

You should consume a variety of vegetables and fruits, with at least 5 servings every day. If you are sensitive to nightshade vegetables, such as tomatoes, potatoes, peppers, and eggplants, you should avoid eating them because they might induce inflammation and increase your digestive issues.

• **Healthy fats include coconut oil, olive oil, avocado, ghee, and animal fats.** These are healthy fat sources that are anti-inflammatory, easy to digest, and full of flavor. You can use them to cook, bake, or season your cuisine.

Coconut oil is especially advantageous since it contains antibacterial qualities that can help battle harmful bacteria and yeast in your gut. Ghee is clarified butter that has been cooked and strained to eliminate milk particles, making it appropriate for dairy-sensitive individuals.

• **Nuts and seeds should be soaked and sprouted**. These are optional, but they can help add crunch, chew, and richness to your cuisine, particularly snacks and sweets. You can also utilize them to make nut and seed butters, milks, flours, and oils that can be used in place of dairy and gluten in recipes.

To minimize antinutrients and enhance digestion, choose raw, unsalted, and organic nuts and seeds, then soak and sprout them before consuming.

You should also avoid nuts and seeds if you are allergic or intolerant to them, or if you have an autoimmune disease, because they might induce inflammation and immunological reactions.

• **Fermented foods include sauerkraut, kimchi, kombucha, and coconut yogurt.** These are probiotic foods that can restore and diversity your gut microbiota, benefiting digestion, immunity, and mood. They can also help create short-chain fatty acids like butyrate and propionate, which can aid in gut healing and inflammation reduction.

You should consume fermented foods on a daily basis, but begin cautiously and gradually increase your intake, as they may induce gas and bloating at first.

If you are allergic to fermented foods or have a histamine sensitivity, you should avoid them because they might trigger allergic responses and headaches.

• **Bone broth, gelatin, and collagen.** These are high in amino acids like glycine, proline, and glutamine, which are necessary for healing and strengthening your gut lining. They also contain minerals such as calcium, magnesium, and phosphorus, which are essential for bone and joint health.

Bone broth should be consumed everyday or used as a foundation for soups and stews. You may also mix gelatin or collagen powder into smoothies, coffee, or tea, or use it to make candies, puddings, or marshmallows.

• **Herbs and spices include ginger, turmeric, garlic, onion, rosemary, thyme, oregano, basil, parsley, cilantro, and others.** These are natural taste enhancers that can make your food both delicious and wholesome.

They also have a variety of health benefits, including improved digestion, reduced inflammation, increased immunity, and ability to fight infections.

Ginger, turmeric, garlic, and onion are particularly effective because to their antibacterial, antifungal, and anti-inflammatory characteristics, which can aid in gut healing. Rosemary, thyme, oregano, basil, parsley, and cilantro are also high in antioxidants, vitamins, and minerals, which can benefit your health.

Foods to Avoid:

• **Grains, including wheat, rice, corn, oats, and quinoa.** These are high in carbohydrates, which can feed harmful bacteria and yeast in your gut, resulting in inflammation and blood sugar increases. They also include gluten, a protein that can harm the gut lining and cause immunological reactions.

They also include anti-nutrients including phytates, lectins, and saponins, which can bind to minerals and inhibit absorption while also irritating the gut lining and causing leaky gut. You should avoid all grains, particularly those containing gluten, such as wheat, barley, rye, and spelt.

You should also avoid pseudo-grains like quinoa, buckwheat, and amaranth, which are technically seeds but have comparable qualities and effects to grains.

• **Legumes include beans, peas, lentils, and soy.** These are high in carbohydrates, which can feed harmful bacteria and yeast in your gut, resulting in inflammation and blood sugar increases.

They also include anti-nutrients including phytates, lectins, and saponins, which can bind to minerals and inhibit absorption while also irritating the gut lining and causing leaky gut. They also contain protease inhibitors, which can disrupt protein digestion and trigger allergies and autoimmune reactions.

You should avoid any legumes, particularly soy, which is highly processed and genetically modified, and can affect hormone and thyroid function.

• **Dairy, including milk, cheese, yogurt, and butter.** These are high in lactose, a sugar that can feed harmful bacteria and yeast in your gut, resulting in inflammation and blood sugar increases. They also include casein, a protein that can irritate the gut lining and cause immunological responses.

They also contain hormones and antibiotics, which can harm your hormones and flora. You should avoid any dairy products, particularly pasteurized and homogenized varieties, which are highly processed and devoid of enzymes and helpful microorganisms.

You should also avoid raw and fermented dairy products like raw milk, cheese, yogurt, and kefir, which are less processed and retain some enzymes and probiotics but still contain lactose and casein, which can trigger allergic responses and infections.

• **Sugars and artificial sweeteners**. These are empty calories that can feed harmful bacteria and yeast in your gut, causing inflammation and blood sugar surges. They may also increase your desires, appetite, and weight gain.

They can also have an impact on your mood, cognitive function, and overall mental health. You should avoid all types of sugar, including table sugar, brown sugar, cane sugar, honey, maple syrup, coconut sugar, agave nectar, and molasses.

You should also avoid artificial sweeteners like aspartame, sucralose, and saccharin, which can alter your gut microbiota and create a variety of health issues.

• **Processed and refined foods include bread, spaghetti, cereal, chips, and cookies**. These are high in toxins, anti-nutrients, and inflammatory compounds, including gluten, sugar, vegetable oils, preservatives, additives, and artificial colors and flavors. They can harm your intestinal lining, create inflammation, and weaken your immune system.

They may also increase your desires, appetite, and weight gain. They can also have an impact on your mood, cognitive function, and overall mental health. You should avoid all processed and refined foods in favor of whole, natural, and unprocessed alternatives.

• **Vegetable oils include canola, soybean, corn, and sunflower oil.** These are high in omega-6 fatty acids, which promote inflammation and oxidative stress in the body. They can also harm your intestinal lining and weaken your immune system.

They can also have an impact on your hormone levels and thyroid function. You should avoid all vegetable oils in favor of healthier fats like coconut oil, olive oil, avocado oil, ghee, and animal fat.

• **Alcohol and caffeine**. These are stimulants and depressants that can interfere with your neurological system, emotions, and sleep. They can also irritate the gut lining, resulting in inflammation and leaky gut.

They can also alter your gut flora, increasing your chances of infection and dysbiosis. They can also impair liver and renal function and detoxification. Avoid or minimize your intake of alcohol and caffeine, and instead go for water, herbal tea, or bone broth.

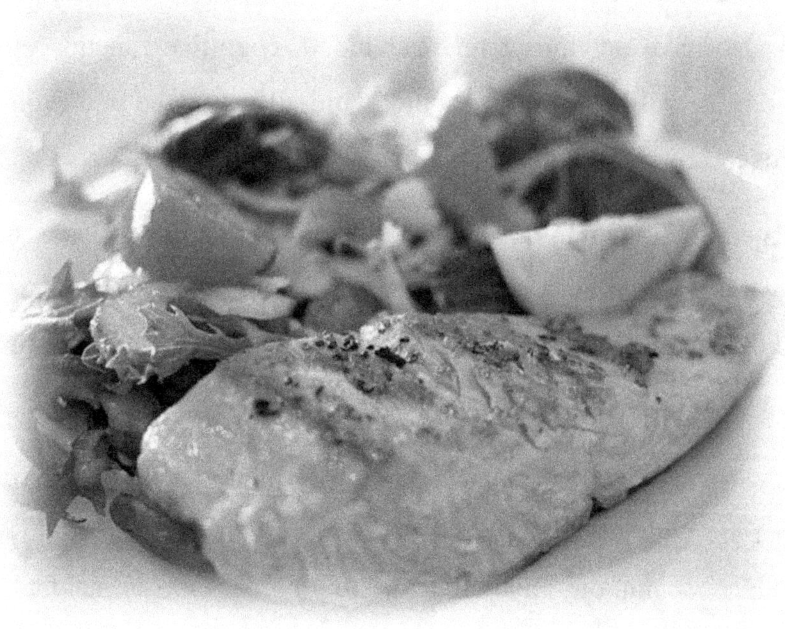

CHAPTER 3

Breakfast Recipes

Coconut Banana Pancakes

- *Servings: four.*
- *Prep time is 10 minutes.*
- *Cook for 15 minutes.*

Ingredients:

- Two ripe bananas, mashed
- 4 eggs, whisked
- One-quarter cup coconut flour
- 1/4 cup unsweetened, shredded coconut
- 1/4 teaspoon of baking soda.
- 1/4 teaspoon of salt.
- One-quarter teaspoon cinnamon
- 2 teaspoons melted coconut oil.
- Serve with honey, maple syrup, or fresh berries (optional).

Instructions:

- In a large mixing basin, add bananas, eggs, coconut flour, shredded coconut, baking soda, salt, and cinnamon. Mix thoroughly until a smooth batter develops.

- Place a big skillet over medium-high heat and coat it with coconut oil. Drop about 1/4 cup batter per pancake into the skillet and cook for 3 minutes, or until bubbles appear on the surface.

- Flip and heat for a further 2 minutes, or until golden and cooked through. Repeat with the remaining batter, using extra coconut oil as needed.

- Serve the pancakes warm, with honey, maple syrup, or fresh berries if desired. Enjoy!

Spinach And Mushroom Frittata

- ***Servings: four.***
- ***Prep time is 10 minutes.***
- ***Cook for 20 minutes.***

Ingredients:

- Eight eggs, beaten
- One-quarter cup almond milk
- 1/4 teaspoon of salt.
- 1/4 teaspoon of black pepper.
- Two tablespoons of ghee or coconut oil.
- 1 onion, chopped
- 2 garlic cloves, minced

- 2 cups sliced mushrooms.
- 4 cups baby spinach, chopped.
- 1/4 cup fresh parsley, chopped

Instructions:

- Preheat the oven to 375°F. Lightly butter a 9-inch pie dish or cast-iron skillet.
- In a medium bowl, combine the eggs, almond milk, salt, and pepper. Set aside.
- In a large skillet over medium-high heat, melt the ghee or coconut oil. Cook the onion and garlic for 10 minutes, stirring periodically, until tender and golden.
- Add the mushrooms and simmer for another 10 minutes, stirring periodically, until browned and soft. Add the spinach and simmer for a few minutes, or until wilted. Stir in the parsley and remove from heat.
- Pour the veggie mixture into the prepared pie dish or pan and spread evenly. Pour the egg mixture over the vegetables, then gently shake the dish or skillet to spread it evenly.
- Bake for 15-20 minutes, or until the frittata is set and brown on top. Allow it to rest for 10 minutes before slicing and serving. Enjoy!

Paleo Granola, Coconut Yogurt, and Berries

- *Servings: four.*
- *Prep time is 10 minutes.*
- *Cook for 20 minutes.*

Ingredients:

- 2 cups raw mixed nuts, including almonds, walnuts, pecans, and cashews.
- 1/4 cup uncooked pumpkin seeds
- 1/4 cup raw sunflower seeds.
- 1/4 cup unsweetened, shredded coconut
- 2 teaspoons melted coconut oil.
- Two tablespoons of honey or maple syrup.
- One teaspoon of vanilla extract.
- One-half teaspoon cinnamon
- 1/4 teaspoon of salt.
- One cup of coconut yogurt.
- 2 cups fresh berries, including strawberries, blueberries, raspberries, and blackberries.

Instructions:

- Preheat the oven to 300°F and prepare a baking sheet using parchment paper or a silicone mat.

- In a food processor or a blender, pulse the nuts until they are finely chopped. Transfer to a large bowl and add the pumpkin seeds, sunflower seeds, shredded coconut, coconut oil, honey or maple syrup, vanilla extract, cinnamon, and salt. Mix thoroughly until everything is well coated.

- Spread the granola mixture evenly on the prepared baking sheet and bake for 15 to 20 minutes, stirring once or twice, until golden and crunchy.

- Let it cool completely on the baking pan before breaking into clusters.

- To serve, divide the coconut yogurt among four bowls and top with the granola and fresh berries. Enjoy!

Bacon and Avocado Egg Muffins

- *Servings: 6*
- *Prep time: 15 minutes*
- *Cook time: 25 minutes*

Ingredients:

- 12 pieces of bacon
- 12 eggs
- Salt and black pepper, to taste
- 1 avocado, peeled and diced

- 2 tablespoons fresh cilantro, chopped
- 1/4 teaspoon cumin
- 1/4 teaspoon paprika
- 1/4 teaspoon garlic powder
- 1/4 teaspoon onion powder
- 1/4 teaspoon of salt.
- 1/4 teaspoon of black pepper.
- 2 tablespoons lime juice

Instructions:

- Preheat the oven to 375°F and grease a 12-cup muffin tray.
- In a large skillet over medium-high heat, fry the bacon until crisp, rotating once, for about 15 minutes. Drain on paper towels and let it cool somewhat.
- Cut each slice into thirds and line each muffin cup with three pieces of bacon, producing a cup shape.
- In a medium bowl, whisk the eggs and season with salt and pepper. Pour the egg mixture equally into each bacon cup, filling about 3/4 full. Bake for 15 to 20 minutes, or until the eggs are set and cooked through.
- In a small bowl, mash the avocado with a fork and add the cilantro, cumin, paprika, garlic powder, onion powder, salt, pepper, and lime juice. Mix well until smooth and creamy.

- To serve, remove the egg muffins from the muffin tray and top with a dollop of the avocado mixture. Enjoy!

Pumpkin Spice Smoothie

- ***Servings: 2***
- ***Prep time: 5 minutes***

Ingredients:

- 1 cup canned pumpkin puree
- 1 cup unsweetened almond milk
- 1/4 cup coconut cream
- Two tablespoons of honey or maple syrup.
- One teaspoon of vanilla extract.
- One-half teaspoon cinnamon
- 1/4 teaspoon nutmeg
- 1/4 teaspoon ginger
- 1/8 teaspoon cloves
- Ice cubes, if needed

Instructions:

- In a blender, combine the pumpkin puree, almond milk, coconut cream, honey or maple syrup, vanilla extract, cinnamon, nutmeg, ginger, and cloves. Blend until smooth and creamy.

- Add ice cubes as needed to modify the thickness and chill the smoothie. Blend again until frothy.
- Pour the smoothie into two glasses and enjoy!

Sweet Potato and Sausage Hash

- *Servings: four.*
- *Prep time: 15 minutes*
- *Cook time: 25 minutes*

Ingredients:

- 4 medium sweet potatoes, peeled and diced
- 2 tablespoons coconut oil, divided
- Salt and black pepper, to taste
- 1 pound ground pork sausage
- 1 onion, chopped
- 2 garlic cloves, minced
- 2 tablespoons dried sage
- 1 teaspoon dried thyme
- 1/4 teaspoon red pepper flakes
- 4 eggs, fried or poached
- Fresh parsley, chopped, for garnish (optional)

Instructions:

- Preheat the oven to 425°F and line a baking sheet with parchment paper or a silicone mat.

- In a large dish, combine the sweet potatoes with 1 tablespoon of coconut oil and season with salt and pepper.

- Spread them equally on the prepared baking sheet and bake for 20 to 25 minutes, or until tender and golden, flipping halfway through.

- In a large skillet over medium-high heat, heat the remaining 1 tablespoon of coconut oil. Add the sausage and simmer, breaking it up with a spatula, for about 15 minutes, or until browned and cooked through.

- Drain the excess grease and transfer the sausage to a platter. Keep warm.

- In the same skillet over medium-high heat, add the onion and garlic and cook, turning regularly, for about 10 minutes, or until soft and golden.

- Add the sage, thyme, red pepper flakes, and salt and pepper to taste and simmer for another 5 minutes, stirring regularly.

- To serve, divide the sweet potato and sausage combination among four dishes and top with an egg and some parsley, if preferred. Enjoy!

Apple Cinnamon Porridge

- *Servings: 2*
- *Prep time: 5 minutes*
- *Cook for 15 minutes.*

Ingredients:

- One-quarter cup coconut flour
- 2 tablespoons flaxseed meal
- 1/4 teaspoon of baking soda.
- 1/4 teaspoon of salt.
- One-quarter teaspoon cinnamon
- 1 1/2 cups unsweetened almond milk
- 1 apple, peeled and grated
- Two tablespoons of honey or maple syrup.
- 2 tablespoons chopped walnuts or pecans

Instructions:

- In a small saucepan over medium heat, stir together the coconut flour, flaxseed meal, baking soda, salt, and cinnamon. Gradually whisk in the almond milk until completely blended and creamy.
- Bring the mixture to a boil, then reduce the heat and simmer, stirring regularly, for about 10 minutes, or until thick and creamy.

- Stir in the apple and honey or maple syrup and cook for another 5 minutes, or until the apple is tender and the porridge is sweetened to your satisfaction.
- Divide the porridge between two bowls and sprinkle with the chopped nuts. Enjoy!

Blueberry Lemon Muffins

- *Servings: 12*
- *Prep time is 10 minutes.*
- *Cook for 20 minutes.*

Ingredients:

- 2 cups almond flour
- One-quarter cup coconut flour
- 1/4 teaspoon of baking soda.
- 1/4 teaspoon of salt.
- 4 eggs
- 1/4 cup coconut oil, melted
- 1/4 cup honey or maple syrup
- 1/4 cup lemon juice
- 2 tablespoons lemon zest
- 1 cup fresh or frozen blueberries

Instructions:

- Preheat the oven to 350°F and line a 12-cup muffin tray with paper liners or oil it thoroughly.
- In a large basin, whisk together the almond flour, coconut flour, baking soda, and salt. In a medium bowl, whisk together the eggs, coconut oil, honey or maple syrup, lemon juice, and lemon zest.
- Add the wet components to the dry ingredients and mix thoroughly until a homogenous batter forms. Fold in the blueberries gently.
- Spoon the batter evenly into the prepared muffin cups, filling about 3/4 full. Bake for 18 to 20 minutes, or until brown and a toothpick inserted in the center comes out clean.
- Let the muffins cool slightly in the tin before transferring to a wire rack to cool completely. Enjoy!

Kale and Onion Quiche

- *Servings: 6*
- *Prep time: 15 minutes*
- *Cook time: 35 minutes*

Ingredients:

• *For the crust:*

- 2 cups almond flour
- 1/4 teaspoon of salt.
- 1/4 cup coconut oil, melted
- 1 egg, beaten

• *For the filling:*

- 1 tablespoon coconut oil
- 1 onion, sliced
- 4 cups kale, chopped and stemmed
- Salt and black pepper, to taste
- 6 eggs
- 1/4 cup unsweetened almond milk
- 1/4 teaspoon nutmeg

Instructions:

- Preheat the oven to 375°F. Lightly butter a 9-inch pie dish or cast-iron skillet.
- In a medium bowl, stir together the almond flour and salt. Add the coconut oil and egg and mix well until a dough forms.
- Press the dough evenly into the bottom and sides of the prepared dish or skillet. Bake for 10 to 12 minutes, or until lightly golden. Set aside.
- In a large skillet over medium-high heat, heat the coconut oil. Add the onion and cook, stirring occasionally, for about 15 minutes, or until soft and caramelized. Add the kale and season with salt and pepper.
- Cook, stirring occasionally, for another 10 minutes, or until wilted and tender. Remove from the heat and spread the mixture over the crust.
- In a medium bowl, whisk together the eggs, almond milk, nutmeg, salt, and pepper. Pour the egg mixture over the kale and onion mixture and gently shake the dish or skillet to distribute it evenly.
- Bake the quiche for 15 to 20 minutes, or until set and golden on top. Allow it to rest for 10 minutes before slicing and serving. Enjoy!

Strawberry Coconut Milkshake

- **Servings: 2**
- **Prep time: 5 minutes**

Ingredients:

- 1 cup canned coconut milk
- 2 cups fresh or frozen strawberries
- Two tablespoons of honey or maple syrup.
- One teaspoon of vanilla extract.
- Ice cubes, if needed

Instructions:

- In a blender, combine the coconut milk, strawberries, honey or maple syrup, and vanilla extract. Blend until smooth and creamy.
- Add ice cubes as needed to adjust the thickness and chill the milkshake. Blend again until frothy.
- Pour the milkshake into two glasses and enjoy!

Chapter 4

Lunch Recipes

Chicken & Vegetable Soup

- *Servings: six.*
- *Prepare time: 15 minutes.*
- *Cook for 30 minutes.*

Ingredients:

- Two tablespoons of coconut oil or ghee.
- 1 onion, chopped
- 2 garlic cloves, minced
- Two carrots, peeled and sliced
- Two celery stalks, chopped
- One teaspoon dried thyme.
- One teaspoon of dried rosemary
- Add salt and black pepper to taste.
- Eight cups of chicken broth.
- 4 cups cooked chicken (shredded or diced)
- Two cups of chopped spinach.
- Fresh parsley, chopped for garnish (optional).

Instructions:

- In a large pot over medium-high heat, melt the coconut oil or ghee. Cook the onion and garlic for about 10 minutes, stirring periodically, until tender and transparent.
- Stir in the carrots, celery, thyme, rosemary, salt, and pepper and simmer for another 10 minutes, or until soft.
- Pour in the chicken broth and heat to a boil. Reduce the heat to a simmer for 10 minutes, or until the flavors are fully blended.
- Cook for another 10 minutes, or until the chicken is thoroughly roasted and the spinach has wilted.
- Serve the soup hot and garnish with parsley if preferred. Enjoy!

Roasted Beet and Kale Salad with Walnuts and Lemon Dressing.

- *Servings: four.*
- *Prepare time: 15 minutes.*
- *Cook for 45 minutes.*

Ingredients:

• *For the Salad:*

- Four medium beets, peeled and chopped

- 2 teaspoons melted coconut oil.

- Add salt and black pepper to taste.

- Eight cups of kale, chopped and stemmed

- 1/4 cup toasted and chopped walnuts.

• For dressing:

- One-quarter cup olive oil

- 2 teaspoons of lemon juice.

- One teaspoon of honey or maple syrup.

- One garlic clove, minced

- Add salt and black pepper to taste.

Instructions:

- Preheat the oven to 400°F and prepare a baking sheet using parchment paper or a silicone mat.

- In a large bowl, combine the beets, coconut oil, salt, and pepper. Spread them equally on the prepared baking sheet and bake for 40 to 45 minutes, or until soft and caramelized. Flip halfway through.

- In a small mixing bowl, combine the olive oil, lemon juice, honey or maple syrup, garlic, salt, and pepper. Set aside.

- In a large skillet over medium-high heat, sauté the kale with a splash of water for 15 minutes, turning periodically, until wilted and soft. Season with salt and pepper to taste.

- To serve, arrange the greens on four plates and top with the roasted beets and walnuts. Drizzle with dressing and enjoy!

Turkey And Apple Lettuce Wraps

- **_Servings: four._**
- **_Prep time is 10 minutes._**
- **_Cook for 15 minutes._**

Ingredients:

- One tablespoon of coconut oil or ghee.
- One pound of ground turkey.
- Add salt and black pepper to taste.
- One-quarter teaspoon garlic powder
- One-quarter teaspoon onion powder
- 1/4 teaspoon of dried sage.
- One-quarter teaspoon dried thyme
- One-quarter teaspoon dried rosemary
- 1/4 cup chopped walnuts.
- One apple, cored and diced
- Two tablespoons of dried cranberries.
- 12 lettuce leaves, including romaine, butter, and iceberg

Instructions:

- In a large skillet over medium-high heat, melt the coconut oil or ghee. Season the turkey with salt, pepper, garlic, onion powder, sage, thyme, and rosemary.

- Cook for approximately 15 minutes, breaking it up with a spatula, or until browned and thoroughly done. Drain the excess grease and place the turkey in a large bowl.

- Toss together the turkey, walnuts, apple, and cranberries.

- To serve, pour a portion of the turkey mixture over each lettuce leaf and wrap it around. Enjoy!

Spicy Tuna Cakes and Avocado Salsa

- *Servings: four.*
- *Prepare time: 15 minutes.*
- *Cook for 15 minutes.*

Ingredients:

• *For the Tuna Cakes:*

- Two cans of drained and flaked tuna.

- Two eggs, beaten

- One-quarter cup almond flour

- 2 teaspoons of chopped fresh cilantro.

- Two tablespoons of chopped fresh parsley

- 2 teaspoons chopped green onion

- One tablespoon of mayonnaise.

- One teaspoon Dijon mustard.

- One teaspoon cumin.

- 1/2 teaspoon paprika.

- 1/4 teaspoon of cayenne pepper.

- Add salt and black pepper to taste.

- Two teaspoons of coconut oil or ghee for frying.

- *For avocado salsa:*

- One ripe avocado, peeled and diced

- 1/4 cup of chopped fresh cilantro.

- 2 tablespoons of chopped red onion.

- Two teaspoons of lime juice.

- Add salt and black pepper to taste.

Instructions:

- In a large bowl, mix together the tuna, eggs, almond flour, cilantro, parsley, green onions, mayonnaise, mustard, cumin, paprika, cayenne, salt, and pepper. Mix thoroughly until a sticky mixture develops. Shape the mixture into eight equal patties and refrigerate for 10 minutes to harden.

- In a small bowl, mash the avocado with a fork, then add the cilantro, onion, lime juice, salt, and pepper. Mix thoroughly until smooth and creamy. Set aside.

- In a large skillet over medium-high heat, melt the coconut oil or ghee. Fry the tuna cakes for 4 minutes on each side, or until golden and crispy. Drain onto paper towels and keep heated.

- To serve, top each tuna cake with some avocado salsa and enjoy!

Cauliflower Rice with Chicken and Broccoli

- *Servings: four.*
- *Prepare time: 15 minutes.*
- *Cook for 20 minutes.*

Ingredients:

- Cut 1 large head of cauliflower into florets.
- Two tablespoons of coconut oil or ghee, split
- Add salt and black pepper to taste.
- Cut 4 chicken breasts into bite-size pieces.
- One-quarter teaspoon garlic powder
- One-quarter teaspoon onion powder
- Four cups broccoli florets.
- One-quarter cup chicken broth
- Two tablespoons of coconut aminos.
- One tablespoon of sesame oil.

- One teaspoon of arrowroot starch.
- Sesame seeds as garnish (optional)

Instructions:

- Using a food processor or blender, pulse the cauliflower florets until they resemble rice. You might need to perform this in batches. Set aside.
- In a large skillet over medium-high heat, melt 1 tablespoon coconut oil or ghee. Season the chicken with salt and pepper, garlic powder, and onion powder.
- Cook, stirring periodically, for approximately 15 minutes, or until browned and cooked through. Transfer to a dish to keep heated.
- Melt the remaining 1 tablespoon coconut oil or ghee in the same skillet over medium-high heat. Cook the broccoli, stirring regularly, for about 10 minutes, or until crisp-tender. Season with salt and pepper to taste.
- In a small bowl, combine the chicken broth, coconut aminos, sesame oil, and arrowroot starch.
- Pour the sauce over the broccoli and heat to a boil. Reduce the heat to a simmer and stir for 5 minutes, or until the sauce thickens.

- To serve, divide the cauliflower rice among four dishes, then top with the chicken and broccoli. Sprinkle with sesame seeds, if preferred. Enjoy!

Creamy Tomato Basil Soup

- *Servings: four.*
- *Prep time is 10 minutes.*
- *Cook for 20 minutes.*

Ingredients:

- Two tablespoons of coconut oil or ghee.
- 1 onion, chopped
- 2 garlic cloves, minced
- Four cups of chicken broth.
- 2 cans diced tomatoes.
- 1/4 cup freshly chopped basil leaves.
- Add salt and black pepper to taste.
- One-quarter cup coconut cream

Instructions:

- In a large pot over medium-high heat, melt the coconut oil or ghee. Cook the onion and garlic for about 10 minutes, stirring periodically, until tender and transparent.

- Bring the soup to a boil by adding the chicken stock, tomatoes, basil, salt, and pepper. Reduce the heat to a simmer for 10 minutes, or until the flavors are fully blended.

- Puree the soup in an immersion blender or normal blender until smooth and creamy. Stir in the coconut cream and adjust the seasoning as needed.

- Serve the soup hot, garnishing with additional basil leaves if desired. Enjoy!

Greek Salad with Chicken and Olives.

- *Servings: four.*
- *Prepare time: 15 minutes.*
- *Cook for 15 minutes.*

Ingredients:

• *For the Salad:*

- Cut 4 chicken breasts into bite-size pieces.
- Two teaspoons of olive oil.
- Add salt and black pepper to taste.
- One teaspoon of dried oregano.
- 8 cups mixed salad greens.
- 1/4 cup of sliced red onion.
- 1/4 cup sliced cucumber.

- 1/4 cup cherry tomatoes, halved

- 1/4 cup pitted Kalamata olives.

• *For dressing:*

- One-quarter cup olive oil

- Two teaspoons of red wine vinegar.

- One tablespoon of lemon juice.

- One garlic clove, minced

- Add salt and black pepper to taste.

Instructions:

- In a large skillet over medium-high heat, heat the olive oil. Season the chicken with salt, pepper, and oregano.

- Cook, stirring periodically, for approximately 15 minutes, or until browned and cooked through. Transfer to a dish to keep heated.

- In a small mixing bowl, combine the olive oil, vinegar, lemon juice, garlic, salt, and pepper. Set aside.

- In a large salad bowl, combine the salad greens and half of the dressing. Divide the salad among four dishes, then top with the chicken, onion, cucumber, tomatoes, and olives. Drizzle with the remaining dressing and enjoy!

Salmon and Cucumber Salad with Dill

- ***Servings: four.***
- ***Prep time is 10 minutes.***
- ***Cook for 15 minutes.***

Ingredients:

- Four salmon fillets, skin on.
- Add salt and black pepper to taste.
- Two tablespoons of coconut oil or ghee.
- Four cups of baby spinach
- Two cups of sliced cucumber.
- 1/4 cup freshly chopped dill.
- 2 teaspoons of lemon juice.
- Two teaspoons of olive oil.

Instructions:

- Preheat the oven to 375°F and prepare a baking sheet using parchment paper or a silicone mat.
- Season the salmon with salt and pepper, then arrange it skin side down on the prepared baking sheet. Bake for 12 to 15 minutes, or until the flesh easily separates with a fork.
- In a large salad bowl, combine the spinach, cucumber, dill, lemon juice, and olive oil. Season with salt and pepper to taste.

- To serve, place the salad on four plates and top with a salmon fillet. Enjoy!

Chicken And Avocado Salad with Lime and Cilantro

- ***Servings: four.***
- ***Prep time is 10 minutes.***
- ***Cook for 15 minutes.***

Ingredients:

- Cut 4 chicken breasts into bite-size pieces.
- Add salt and black pepper to taste.
- Two tablespoons of coconut oil or ghee.
- Four cups mixed salad greens.
- Two avocados, peeled and diced
- 1/4 cup of chopped fresh cilantro.
- Two teaspoons of lime juice.
- Two teaspoons of olive oil.
- One-quarter teaspoon cumin
- One-quarter teaspoon garlic powder

Instructions:

- In a large skillet over medium-high heat, melt the coconut oil or ghee. Season the chicken with salt and pepper, cumin, and garlic powder.

- Cook, stirring periodically, for approximately 15 minutes, or until browned and cooked through. Transfer to a dish to keep heated.

- In a small bowl, combine the lime juice and olive oil. Set aside.

- In a large salad bowl, combine the salad greens and half of the dressing. Divide the salad among four dishes, then top with the chicken and avocado.

- Garnish with cilantro and sprinkle with the remaining dressing. Enjoy!

Roasted Butternut Squash and Apple Soup

- *Servings: four.*
- *Prepare time: 15 minutes.*
- *Cook for 45 minutes.*

Ingredients:

- One large butternut squash, peeled and cubed
- Two apples, cored and cut

- 2 teaspoons melted coconut oil.

- Add salt and black pepper to taste.

- Four cups of chicken broth.

- 1/4 teaspoon nutmeg.

- One-quarter teaspoon cinnamon

- One-quarter cup coconut cream

- Fresh parsley, chopped for garnish (optional).

Instructions:

- Preheat the oven to 400°F and prepare a baking sheet using parchment paper or a silicone mat.

- In a large mixing bowl, combine the squash and apple with the coconut oil and season with salt and pepper.

- Spread them equally on the prepared baking sheet and bake for 35 to 40 minutes, or until soft and caramelized. Flip halfway through.

- Heat the chicken stock in a large pot over medium-high heat until it boils. Simmer for 10 minutes, or until the flavors are well mixed.

- Puree the soup in an immersion blender or normal blender until smooth and creamy. Stir in the coconut cream and adjust the seasoning as needed.

- Serve the soup hot and garnish with parsley if preferred. Enjoy!

CHAPTER 5

<u>*Dinner Recipes*</u>

<u>*Beef and Vegetable Stew*</u>

- *Servings: six.*
- *Prepare time: 15 minutes.*
- *Cooking time: four hours.*

Ingredients:

- Two teaspoons of coconut oil.
- Cut 2 pounds of beef chuck into 1-inch cubes.
- Salt and pepper to taste.
- 1 onion, chopped
- 4 garlic cloves, minced
- Two tablespoons of tomato paste.
- Four cups of beef broth.
- Two bay leaves.
- One teaspoon dried thyme.
- One teaspoon of dried rosemary.
- 4 peeled and sliced carrots.
- Two celery stalks, chopped
- Two parsnips, peeled and sliced
- 1/4 cup arrowroot starch.

- One-quarter cup water
- Fresh parsley (for garnish)

Instructions:

- Cook the coconut oil in a large skillet over medium-high heat. Season the beef with salt and pepper, then brown on all sides for about 15 minutes. Transfer to the slow cooker.
- Cook the onion, garlic, and tomato paste in the same skillet, stirring, until tender, about 10 minutes.
- Bring the broth, bay leaves, thyme, and rosemary to a boil. Pour the mixture onto the beef in the slow cooker.
- Stir the carrots, celery, and parsnips into the slow cooker until well combined. Cover and simmer on low for 4 hours, or until the beef is cooked.
- In a small bowl, combine the arrowroot starch and water. Stir into the stew and heat on high for 15 minutes, or until slightly thickened.
- Sprinkle with parsley and serve.

Salmon With Asparagus with Lemon and Dill.

- *Servings: four.*
- *Prep time is 10 minutes.*
- *Cook for 15 minutes.*

Ingredients:

- 4 salmon fillets, approximately 6 ounces each.
- Salt and pepper to taste.
- Two tablespoons of ghee.
- Two lemons: one cut and one juiced
- 2 tablespoons fresh dill, chopped
- One pound of trimmed asparagus

Instructions:

- Preheat the oven to 425°F. Line a baking sheet with parchment paper. Season the salmon with salt and pepper, then set it on the prepared baking sheet.
- Dot with ghee, then top with lemon slices and half of the dill. Bake for 12–15 minutes, or until the salmon is flaky and cooked through.
- Meanwhile, cook the asparagus in a steamer basket over boiling water for about 10 minutes, or until crisp-tender. Drizzle with lemon juice and add the remaining dill. Season with salt and pepper to taste.

- Serve the fish alongside the asparagus and enjoy.

Roasted Chicken with Root Vegetables and Rosemary.

- *Servings: four.*
- *Prepare time: 15 minutes.*
- *Cooking time: one hour.*

Ingredients:

- 1 entire chicken, approximately 4 pounds.
- Salt and pepper to taste.
- 4 tablespoons of melted ghee.
- Four fresh sprigs of rosemary
- 4 cloves of garlic, peeled and mashed
- Four medium carrots, peeled and cut into bits
- 4 medium parsnips, peeled and chopped into bits
- Two medium turnips, peeled and sliced into wedges
- 1 large onion peeled and sliced into wedges

Instructions:

- Preheat the oven to 375°F. Lightly oil a baking dish with ghee. Rinse the chicken, then blot it dry with paper towels.

Season the cavity with salt and pepper, then stuff it with 2 sprigs of rosemary and 2 cloves garlic.

- Tie the legs together with kitchen twine, then tuck the wings under the torso. Place the chicken in the prepared baking dish and brush with half of the melted ghee.

- Season the skin with salt and pepper and arrange the remaining rosemary and garlic around the bird.

- In a large mixing bowl, combine the root vegetables and onion with the remaining ghee and season with salt and pepper. Arrange in a single layer around the bird. Roast for 1 hour, or until the chicken is golden and fully cooked, and the vegetables are soft. Baste the chicken and vegetables with the pan juices midway through the cooking process.

- Place the chicken on a chopping board and let it rest for 10 minutes before slicing. Serve with roasted vegetables and enjoy.

<u>Spaghetti Squash with Meatballs and Tomato Sauce</u>

- *Servings: four.*
- *Prepare time: 15 minutes.*
- *Cook for 45 minutes.*

Ingredients:

- 1 large spaghetti squash halved and seeded.
- Two teaspoons of coconut oil.
- Salt and pepper to taste.
- One pound of ground beef.
- One-quarter cup almond flour
- One egg, lightly beaten
- 2 teaspoons Italian seasoning.
- One-quarter teaspoon of garlic powder
- One-quarter teaspoon of onion powder
- Two cups of tomato sauce.
- Fresh basil for garnish.

Instructions:

- Preheat the oven to 400°F. Line a baking sheet with parchment paper. Rub 1 tablespoon coconut oil onto the cut sides of the spaghetti squash and season with salt and pepper.

- Place the squash, cut side down, on the prepared baking sheet and bake for 35 to 40 minutes, until soft.
- In a large bowl, mix together the ground beef, almond flour, egg, Italian seasoning, garlic powder, onion powder, salt, and pepper.
- Mix thoroughly and shape into 16 meatballs. Heat the remaining coconut oil in a large skillet over medium-high heat. Cook the meatballs for 15 to 20 minutes, rotating regularly, until they are browned and cooked through.
- Drain the excess fat, then add the tomato sauce. Simmer for ten minutes, or until slightly thickened.
- Using a fork, scrape the spaghetti squash strands into a large bowl. Serve with the meatballs and sauce, garnished with basil.

<u>Thai Coconut Curry with Shrimp and Zucchini Noodles.</u>

- *Servings: four.*
- *Prepare time: 15 minutes.*
- *Cook for 15 minutes.*

Ingredients:

- Four medium zucchinis spiralized or peeled into thin noodles.
- Salt to taste.
- Two teaspoons of coconut oil.
- One pound of big shrimp, peeled and deveined
- 1/4 cup chopped green onions.
- 2 tablespoons of minced ginger.
- 2 garlic cloves, minced
- 1/4 teaspoon red pepper flakes.
- One 14-ounce can of full-fat coconut milk.
- 2 tablespoons red curry paste.
- Two teaspoons of lime juice.
- Two teaspoons of fish sauce.
- Fresh cilantro for garnish.

Instructions:

- Place the zucchini noodles in a colander over a large basin and season with salt. Allow them to drain for 10 minutes, then squeeze out any extra water with your hands or a clean towel.

- Cook the coconut oil in a large skillet over medium-high heat. Cook the shrimp for 6 to 8 minutes, stirring once, until pink and cooked through. Transfer to a dish to keep heated.

- In the same skillet, combine the green onions, ginger, garlic, and red pepper flakes. Cook for 2 minutes, stirring, or until aromatic.

- Bring the coconut milk, curry paste, lime juice, and fish sauce to a boil. Reduce the heat to a simmer for 10 minutes, or until slightly thickened.

- Add the zucchini noodles and toss to coat in the sauce. Cook for 5 minutes, or until well cooked and tender. Serve beside the shrimp, garnished with cilantro.

Lamb & Eggplant Moussaka

- *Servings: six.*
- *Prep time is 20 minutes.*
- *Cook for 40 minutes.*

Ingredients:

- 2 large eggplants, cut into 1/4-inch-thick rounds.
- Salt to taste.
- Two teaspoons of coconut oil.
- 1 onion, chopped
- 4 garlic cloves, minced
- One pound of ground lamb.
- Two teaspoons of dried oregano.
- One teaspoon of cinnamon.
- 1/4 teaspoon nutmeg.
- 1/4 teaspoon black pepper.
- One fifteen-ounce can of tomato sauce.
- 2 eggs
- One-quarter cup coconut milk
- Two tablespoons of nutritional yeast.

Instructions:

- Preheat the oven to 375°F and gently butter a 9-by-13-inch baking dish. Sprinkle the eggplant slices with salt and allow to set for 15 minutes before patting them dry with paper towels.

- Cook the coconut oil in a large skillet over medium-high heat. Stir in the onion and garlic and simmer for 10 minutes, or until tender.

- Add the lamb, oregano, cinnamon, nutmeg, pepper, and 1/2 teaspoon salt and simmer for 15 minutes, breaking up the meat with a spatula, until browned and cooked through.

- Stir in the tomato sauce and cook for 10 minutes, or until slightly thickened.

- In a small bowl, combine the eggs, coconut milk, and nutritional yeast. Season with salt and pepper to taste.

- Place half of the eggplant slices in a single layer on the bottom of the prepared baking dish. Spread the lamb mixture over the eggplant evenly.

- Top with the remaining eggplant pieces and pour the egg mixture over top. Bake for 25–30 minutes, or until brown and bubbling.

- Allow the moussaka to rest for ten minutes before serving.

Chicken & Mushroom Casserole

- *Servings: four.*
- *Prep time is 10 minutes.*
- *Cook for 35 minutes.*

Ingredients:

- Four boneless, skinless chicken breasts.
- Salt and pepper to taste.
- Two tablespoons of ghee.
- 1 onion, chopped
- 4 garlic cloves, minced
- Eight ounces of chopped mushrooms
- Two tablespoons of arrowroot starch.
- Two cups of chicken broth.
- One-quarter cup coconut cream
- 2 tablespoons fresh parsley, chopped

Instructions:

- Preheat the oven to 375°F and gently butter a 9-by-13-inch baking dish. Season the chicken with salt and pepper before placing it in the prepared baking dish.
- Melt the ghee in a large skillet over medium-high heat. Stir in the onion and garlic and simmer for 10 minutes, or until tender.

- Stir in the mushrooms and simmer for another 10 minutes, or until browned and soft. Sprinkle the arrowroot starch over the mushroom mixture and stir well.

- Bring the chicken broth to a boil, whisking in gradually. Reduce the heat to a simmer for 10 minutes, or until slightly thickened. Add the coconut cream and parsley, and season to taste with salt and pepper.

- Pour the mushroom sauce over the chicken and bake for 15-20 minutes, or until the chicken is fully cooked and the sauce is bubbling.

- Enjoy the chicken and mushroom casserole.

Baked Cod with Lemon and Capers

- *Servings: four.*
- *Prep time is 10 minutes.*
- *Cook for 15 minutes.*

Ingredients:

- 4 fish fillets, approximately 6 ounces each.
- Salt and pepper to taste.
- 2 tablespoons of melted ghee.
- Two teaspoons of lemon juice.
- 2 tablespoons capers, drained

- 2 tablespoons fresh parsley, chopped

Instructions:

- Preheat the oven to 400°F. Lightly oil a baking dish with ghee. Season the fish with salt and pepper before placing it in the prepared baking dish.
- In a small bowl, combine the ghee, lemon juice, and capers. Pour over the cod and bake for 12 to 15 minutes, or until readily flaked with a fork.
- Sprinkle with parsley and serve.

Moroccan Beef & Apricot Tagine

- **Servings: six.**
- **Prepare time: 15 minutes.**
- **Cooking time: four hours.**

Ingredients:

- Two teaspoons of coconut oil.
- Cut 2 pounds of beef chuck into 1-inch cubes.
- Salt and pepper to taste.
- 1 onion, chopped
- 4 garlic cloves, minced
- Two teaspoons of cumin.
- Two teaspoons of paprika.

- One teaspoon of cinnamon.

- 1/4 teaspoon cayenne pepper.

- Four cups of beef broth.

- 1/4 cup dried apricots, chopped

- 2 tablespoons fresh cilantro, chopped

Instructions:

- Cook the coconut oil in a large skillet over medium-high heat. Season the beef with salt and pepper, then brown on all sides for about 15 minutes. Transfer to the slow cooker.

- Cook the onion, garlic, cumin, paprika, cinnamon, and cayenne pepper in the same skillet, stirring, until tender, about 10 minutes.

- Bring the broth to a boil. Pour the mixture onto the beef in the slow cooker.

- Stir in the apricots until thoroughly combined. Cover and simmer on low for 4 hours, or until the beef is cooked.

- Garnish with cilantro and serve.

Roasted Cauliflower with Garlic Soup

- *Servings: four.*
- *Prepare time: 15 minutes.*
- *Cook for 45 minutes.*

Ingredients:

- Cut 1 large head of cauliflower into florets.
- 1/4 cup melted coconut oil.
- Salt and pepper to taste.
- 1 garlic bulb with top chopped off
- Four cups of chicken broth.
- One-quarter cup coconut cream
- 2 teaspoons of freshly chopped chives.

Instructions:

- Preheat the oven to 425°F. Line a baking sheet with parchment paper. Toss the cauliflower with 2 tablespoons coconut oil and season with salt and pepper.
- Spread out in a single layer on the prepared baking sheet. Drizzle the remaining coconut oil over the garlic bulb, then wrap it in foil.
- Place on the same baking sheet as the cauliflower. Roast for 25–30 minutes, or until the cauliflower is golden and the garlic is tender.

- Squeeze the roasted garlic cloves from their skins and put to a blender. Add half of the roasted cauliflower and half of the chicken broth, then mix until smooth.

- Transfer the mixture to a large pot, and repeat with the remaining cauliflower and broth.

- Bring the soup to a boil, then reduce the heat and let it simmer for 15 minutes, or until somewhat thicker. Add the coconut cream and season with salt and pepper to taste.

- Ladle the soup into dishes and sprinkle with chives. Enjoy the roasted cauliflower and garlic soup.

CHAPTER 6

<u>*Snack and Dessert Recipes*</u>

<u>*Almond Butter and Banana Bites*</u>

- *Servings: 4*
- *Prep time: 10 minutes*

Ingredients:

- Two ripe bananas, cut
- One-quarter cup almond butter
- Two tablespoons of dark chocolate chips.
- One teaspoon of coconut oil.

Instructions:

- Line a baking sheet with parchment paper and put the banana slices in a single layer. Place a spoonful of almond butter on each slice and freeze for 15 minutes, or until firm.
- In a small microwave-safe bowl, mix together the chocolate chips and coconut oil. Microwave for 30 seconds, or until completely melted, stirring every 10 seconds.
- Drizzle the chocolate over the banana bites, then freeze for another 10 minutes, or until set.
- Enjoy almond butter and banana pieces as a snack or dessert.

<u>*Carrot Cake Energy Balls.*</u>

- ***Serves: 16***
- ***Prepare time: 15 minutes.***

Ingredients:

- One cup shredded carrot.
- One cup of pitted dates.
- 1/2 cup unsweetened shredded coconut, plus extra for rolling.
- 1/4 cup raw cashews.
- Two tablespoons of almond butter.
- One teaspoon of vanilla extract.
- 1/2 teaspoon cinnamon.
- 1/4 teaspoon nutmeg.
- 1/8 teaspoon salt.

Instructions:

- Place the carrots in a food processor and pulse until finely chopped. Process the dates, coconut, cashews, almond butter, vanilla, cinnamon, nutmeg, and salt until a sticky dough forms.
- Scoop out tablespoon-sized bits of dough and roll them into balls.

- Coat with more shredded coconut if preferred and place on a parchment-lined baking sheet. Refrigerate for at least 1 hour, or until firm.
- Eat carrot cake energy balls as a snack or dessert.

Paleo Chocolate Chip Cookies.

- ***Serves: 12***
- ***Prep time: 10 minutes***
- ***Cook for 10 minutes.***

Ingredients:

- 1/4 cup melted coconut oil.
- One-quarter cup maple syrup
- 1 egg
- One teaspoon of vanilla extract.
- Two cups of almond flour.
- One-half teaspoon of baking soda
- One-quarter teaspoon of salt
- One-quarter cup dark chocolate chips

Instructions:

- Preheat the oven to 350°F. Line a baking sheet with parchment paper. In a large mixing basin, blend the coconut

- oil, maple syrup, egg, and vanilla until thoroughly incorporated.
- In a larger basin, combine the almond flour, baking soda, and salt. Combine the dry ingredients with the wet components and whisk until a dough forms. Fold in the chocolate chips.
- Drop by rounded tablespoonfuls onto the prepared baking sheet, leaving some space between each.
- Flatten slightly with your fingers or a spatula. Bake for 10–12 minutes, or until brown and firm.
- Treat your paleo chocolate chip cookies as a snack or dessert.

Coconut And Berry Popsicles

- *Servings: six.*
- *Prep time: 10 minutes*
- *Freeze time: four hours.*

Ingredients:

- 2 cups fresh or frozen mixed berries.
- One-quarter cup water
- Two teaspoons of honey.
- One 14-ounce can of full-fat coconut milk.
- One teaspoon of vanilla extract.

Instructions:

- In a small saucepan over medium heat, combine the berries, water, and honey. Bring to a boil, then reduce heat and cook for 10 minutes, or until the berries are soft and syrupy. Mash with a fork or a potato masher and allow to cool somewhat.

- In a medium bowl, combine the coconut milk and vanilla. Spoon part of the berry mixture into popsicle Molds, about 1/4 full.

- Pour part of the coconut mixture over the berries, filling them about 1/4 of the way. Repeat with the remaining berry and coconut mixes, alternately layering until the Molds are full. Insert the popsicle sticks and freeze for at least 4 hours, or until firm.

- Eat your coconut and berry popsicles as a snack or dessert.

Apple and Cinnamon Muffins

- *Serves: 12*
- *Prepare time: 15 minutes.*
- *Cook time: 20 minutes*

Ingredients:

- Two cups of almond flour.
- One-quarter cup coconut flour

- 2 tablespoons baking soda.

- One-quarter teaspoon of salt

- Two teaspoons of cinnamon.

- 1/4 teaspoon nutmeg.

- 4 eggs

- 1/4 cup melted coconut oil.

- One-quarter cup maple syrup

- One teaspoon of vanilla extract.

- 1 1/2 cups shredded apple.

Instructions:

- Preheat the oven to 350°F. Line a muffin tray with paper liners. In a large basin, combine the almond flour, coconut flour, baking soda, salt, cinnamon, and nutmeg.

- In a medium bowl, combine the eggs, coconut oil, maple syrup, and vanilla. Stir the wet and dry ingredients together until thoroughly blended. Fold in the grated apples.

- Scoop the batter into the prepared muffin tray, filling each cup about 3/4 full. Bake for 18 to 20 minutes, or until a toothpick inserted in the center comes out clean.

- Enjoy your apple and cinnamon muffins as a snack or dessert.

Pumpkin Pie Bars

- *Serves: 16*
- *Prepare time: 15 minutes.*
- *Cook for 35 minutes.*

Ingredients:

• *For the crust:*

- Two cups of almond flour.
- 1/4 cup melted coconut oil.
- 2 teaspoons of maple syrup
- One-quarter teaspoon of salt

• *For the filling:*

- 1 15-ounce can of pumpkin puree
- One-quarter cup coconut milk
- 3 eggs
- One-quarter cup maple syrup
- 2 tablespoons of pumpkin pie spice
- One-quarter teaspoon of salt

Instructions:

- Preheat the oven to 350°F and gently butter a 9x9-inch baking dish. In a medium bowl, stir together the almond flour, coconut oil, maple syrup, and salt until a crumbly dough forms.

- Press the dough evenly into the bottom and slightly up the sides of the prepared baking dish. Bake for 10 minutes, or until lightly golden.

- In a large bowl, whisk together the pumpkin puree, coconut milk, eggs, maple syrup, pumpkin pie spice, and salt until smooth and well combined.

- Pour the filling over the crust and spread it evenly. Bake for 25 to 30 minutes, or until the filling is set and the edges are slightly browned.

- Let the bars cool completely on a wire rack, then refrigerate for at least 2 hours, or until firm. Cut into 16 squares and enjoy your pumpkin pie bars as a snack or dessert.

Coconut Macaroons

- *Servings: 24*
- *Prep time: 10 minutes*
- *Cook time: 15 minutes*

Ingredients:

- 3 cups of unsweetened shredded coconut
- 1/4 cup of honey

- 2 egg whites
- One-quarter teaspoon of salt
- 1/4 teaspoon of vanilla extract

Instructions:

- Preheat the oven to 350°F. Line a baking sheet with parchment paper. In a large basin, stir the coconut with the honey until well coated.
- In a larger bowl, whisk the egg whites with the salt and vanilla until stiff peaks form. Gently incorporate the egg whites into the coconut mixture until completely mixed.
- Drop by rounded tablespoonfuls onto the prepared baking sheet, leaving some space between each.
- Bake for 12 to 15 minutes, or until golden and crisp on the edges.
- Enjoy your coconut macaroons as a snack or dessert.

Chocolate Avocado Pudding

- *Servings: 4*
- *Prep time: 10 minutes*

Ingredients:

- 2 ripe avocados, peeled and pitted
- 1/4 cup of raw cacao powder

- One-quarter cup maple syrup
- One-quarter cup coconut milk
- One teaspoon of vanilla extract.
- A pinch of salt

Instructions:

- In a blender or food processor, add all the ingredients and blend until smooth and creamy, scraping down the sides as needed.
- Transfer the pudding to a bowl and refrigerate for at least an hour, or until cooled and hard.
- Enjoy your chocolate avocado pudding as a snack or dessert.

Lemon and Ginger Gummies

- *Servings: 24*
- *Prep time: 10 minutes*
- *Cook for 5 minutes.*

Ingredients:

- A quarter cup of fresh lemon juice
- 2 teaspoons grated ginger.
- One-quarter cup water
- Three teaspoons of gelatin.
- Two teaspoons of honey.

Instructions:

- In a small saucepan over low heat, combine the lemon juice, ginger, water, gelatin, and honey.

- Whisk until smooth. Bring to a boil, then cook for 5 minutes, stirring regularly.

- Transfer the mixture to a silicone Mold or an 8x8-inch baking dish lined with parchment paper. Refrigerate for at least two hours, or until set.

- Cut the lemon and ginger candies into small squares or pop them out of the Mold to enjoy as a snack or dessert.

Paleo Brownies

- ***Serves: 16***
- ***Prep time is 10 minutes.***
- ***Cook for 25 minutes.***

Ingredients:

- 1/2 cup melted coconut oil.
- One-half cup raw honey
- 2 eggs
- One teaspoon of vanilla extract.
- 1/2 cup almond flour.
- 1/2 cup raw cacao powder.

- One-quarter teaspoon of baking soda

- One-quarter teaspoon of salt

- One-quarter cup dark chocolate chips

Instructions:

- Preheat the oven to 350°F, then gently coat an 8x8-inch baking dish with coconut oil. In a large mixing bowl, add the coconut oil, honey, eggs, and vanilla until well blended.

- In a medium bowl, combine almond flour, cacao powder, baking soda, and salt. Mix the dry ingredients into the wet components until completely blended. Fold in the chocolate chips.

- Pour the batter into the prepared baking dish and spread evenly. Bake for 20–25 minutes, or until a toothpick inserted in the center comes out clean.

- Eat paleo brownies as a snack or dessert.

14-day Paleo Gut Healing Meal Plan

Day 1

- Breakfast: Coconut Banana Pancakes.
- Lunch: Chicken and vegetable soup.
- Dinner: Beef and vegetable stew.
- Snack/dessert: Almond butter and banana bites.

Day 2

- Breakfast: Spinach and mushroom frittata
- Lunch: Roasted beet and kale salad with walnuts and lemon dressing.
- Dinner is salmon and asparagus with lemon and dill.
- Snack or dessert: Carrot Cake Energy Balls.

Day 3

- Breakfast: Paleo granola with coconut yogurt and berries.
- Lunch: turkey and apple lettuce wraps.
- Dinner: Roasted chicken with root vegetables and rosemary.
- Snack or Dessert: Paleo Chocolate Chip Cookies.

Day 4

- Breakfast: Bacon and avocado egg muffins.
- Lunch: Spicy Tuna Cakes and Avocado Salsa
- Dinner is spaghetti squash with meatballs and tomato sauce.
- Snack/dessert: Coconut and Berry Popsicles.

Day 5

- Breakfast: Pumpkin Spice Smoothie.
- Lunch: Cauliflower rice with chicken and broccoli.
- Dinner: Thai Coconut Curry with Shrimp and Zucchini noodles.
- Snack or dessert: Apple and Cinnamon Muffins.

Day 6

- Breakfast: Sweet potato and sausage hash.
- Lunch: Creamy tomato and basil soup.
- Dinner: Lamb and Eggplant Moussaka.
- Snack or Dessert: Pumpkin Pie Bars.

Day 7

- Breakfast: Apple Cinnamon Porridge.
- Lunch: Greek salad with chicken and olives.
- Dinner is Chicken and Mushroom Casserole.
- Snack or Dessert: Coconut Macaroons

Day 8

- Breakfast: blueberry lemon muffins.

- Lunch: Salmon and cucumber salad with dill.

- Dinner: Baked cod with lemon and capers.

- Snack or Dessert: Chocolate Avocado Pudding

Day 9

- Breakfast: Kale and onion quiche

- Lunch: Chicken and avocado salad with lime and cilantro.

- Dinner: Moroccan Beef with Apricot Tagine.

- Snack or dessert: Lemon and Ginger Gummies

Day 10

- Breakfast: strawberry coconut milkshake.

- Lunch: Roasted Butternut Squash with Apple Soup

- Dinner: Roasted cauliflower and garlic soup.

- Snack or Dessert: Paleo Brownies

Day 11

- Breakfast: Coconut Banana Pancakes.

- Lunch: Chicken and vegetable soup.

- Dinner is salmon and asparagus with lemon and dill.

- Snack/dessert: Almond butter and banana bites.

Day 12

- Breakfast: Spinach and mushroom frittata
- Lunch: Roasted beet and kale salad with walnuts and lemon dressing.
- Dinner: Roasted chicken with root vegetables and rosemary.
- Snack or dessert: Carrot Cake Energy Balls.

Day 13

- Breakfast: Paleo granola with coconut yogurt and berries.
- Lunch: turkey and apple lettuce wraps.
- Dinner is spaghetti squash with meatballs and tomato sauce.
- Snack or Dessert: Paleo Chocolate Chip Cookies.

Day 14

- Breakfast: Bacon and avocado egg muffins.
- Lunch: Spicy Tuna Cakes and Avocado Salsa
- Dinner: Thai Coconut Curry with Shrimp and Zucchini noodles.
- Snack/dessert: Coconut and Berry Popsicles.

I hope you loved the 14-day paleo gut healing meal plan.

CONCLUSION

You've finished this book, and I hope you liked reading it and learning about the paleo gut healing diet. This diet is intended to help you restore gut health, improve digestion, decrease inflammation, and improve your general well-being. By following the ideas and recipes in this book, you can get the benefits of eating natural, nutritious, and nutrient-dense foods that nourish both your body and mind.

However, this book is not intended to replace professional medical advice, diagnosis, or treatment. Everyone's health situation is unique, and you may have special demands or circumstances that necessitate personalized care.

As a result, I strongly recommend that you contact with your healthcare provider before beginning or changing any diet or lifestyle regimen. They can assist you in assessing your objectives, tracking your progress, and addressing any potential challenges or concerns along the road.

I also invite you to share your thoughts and experiences with me and the other readers. Your opinion is very important to me, and I would love to hear from you. Please give a positive review and let me know what you enjoyed, learned, and accomplished. I am excited to hear your success stories and help you on your path to maximum health.

Thank you for selecting this book and entrusting me as your guide. I hope you found it interesting, useful, and enjoyable. Remember, you are what you eat, so eat wisely and live well.

I Wish You All the Best on Your Paleo Gut Healing Adventure

www.ingramcontent.com/pod-product-compliance
Lightning Source LLC
Chambersburg PA
CBHW050819250726
48653CB00006B/2313